GALLSTONE DIET FOR WOMEN OVER 40

Delicious Recipes to Maintain a Healthy Gallbladder, Control Your Weight, and Look Fabulous at Forty and Beyond

DR LANA BROWN, RN

Copyright Page

© 2024 by Dr. Lana Brown.

For permissions requests, write to the author at www.thelanabrown.com

Table of Contents

INTRODUCTION

Gallstones are pieces of solid material that form in your gallbladder, a small organ located under your liver. This condition is known as cholelithiasis. Your gallbladder stores and releases bile, a fluid made by your liver, which helps with digestion. Bile also carries cholesterol and wastes like bilirubin, a byproduct of red blood cell breakdown. Gallstones form when these substances are out of balance.

Gallstones can be as small as a grain of sand or as large as a golf ball. You might have one large stone or many small ones, and sometimes a mix of both. Often, you won't know you have gallstones unless they block a bile duct, causing pain. Most gallstones don't cause symptoms or health problems. These "silent gallstones" usually don't need treatment. However, if you experience sudden and severe pain that lasts for hours, seek medical help immediately, as it can be a sign that gallstones are blocking your bile duct, which can be life-threatening.

There are two main types of gallstones: cholesterol stones and pigment stones. Cholesterol stones are typically yellow-green and are primarily made of undissolved cholesterol, although they can contain other substances like bilirubin or bile salts. These are the most common, accounting for about 80% of gallstones. Pigment stones are brown or black and consist mostly of bilirubin. They are more common in people with liver disease or blood disorders like sickle cell anemia or leukemia.

You can have gallstones without knowing it. Symptoms usually occur only when gallstones block the flow of bile from your gallbladder to your small intestine, a condition known as a gallbladder attack or biliary colic. Symptoms include pain in the upper right side of your abdomen just under your ribs, pain in your lower chest, right shoulder, or back, an upset stomach, nausea or vomiting, and other digestive issues like indigestion, heartburn, and gas.

Gallstones may pass on their own, but sometimes immediate medical care is necessary. You should see your doctor or go to the hospital if your belly pain lasts more than two hours or is severe, if you have a fever with chills, or if your skin or eyes turn yellow. Not treating gallstones promptly can lead to complications such as infection and inflammation. It's crucial to talk to your doctor because a gallbladder attack can mimic other conditions that also require treatment, such as appendicitis, ulcers, or pancreatitis.

CHAPTER I

UNDERSTANDING GALLSTONES

Gallstones, which are small stones typically composed of cholesterol, can pose unique challenges for women over 40. These stones form in the gallbladder, a small organ beneath the liver responsible for storing and concentrating bile—a substance essential for digesting fats. While many individuals with gallstones experience no symptoms, the situation can be quite different for those who do, particularly women in this age group.

For women over 40, gallstones can lead to sudden, intense abdominal pain known as biliary colic. This discomfort usually lasts from one to five hours and often originates in the upper right abdomen, under the ribcage. However, it can also radiate to other areas, including the right arm, shoulder, back, or even the chest. This radiation of pain might be more pronounced in women, potentially leading to confusion with other conditions such as heartburn or, in some cases, heart attacks.

One key aspect for women in this demographic is their increased tendency to experience referred pain. This means that the pain from gallstones may be felt in areas other than where the problem originates. For instance, pain might be perceived in the arm, shoulder, or chest, which can complicate diagnosis and management. Additionally, women over 40 are more prone to chronic pain and might be inclined to dismiss intermittent pain as mere discomfort or indigestion.

Complications from gallstones can also arise, such as cholecystitis, or inflammation of the gallbladder. Given the natural tendency for pain to be more diffused or less straightforward in women, it becomes essential for those experiencing severe or recurring pain to seek medical attention promptly. Gallstone attacks are often recurrent, so early intervention can be crucial in managing symptoms and preventing further complications.

Understanding these nuances is important for women over 40 to ensure they can effectively recognize symptoms and seek appropriate care. Balancing awareness of symptoms with proactive health management can make a significant difference in their quality of life and overall well-being.

Causes Risk Factors Symptoms and Complications

Gallstones are small, cholesterol-based stones that can form in the gallbladder, a crucial organ for storing and concentrating bile produced by the liver. For women over 40, the risk and impact of gallstones are particularly notable due to several interconnected factors. As women age, their risk of developing gallstones increases, partly due to hormonal changes that can affect bile composition and gallbladder function. Additionally, women are more prone to experiencing referred pain from gallstones, which can make the diagnosis more challenging.

Causes and Risk Factors

Gallstones form when there is an imbalance in the substances that make up bile, such as cholesterol. For women over 40, several risk factors can contribute to this imbalance. Hormonal changes associated with aging, including menopause, can alter cholesterol levels in bile, increasing the likelihood of gallstone formation. Being female and having a family history of gallstones further heightens the risk. Other contributing factors include inflammatory bowel disease, rapid weight loss of more than 1.5 kg per week, and weight loss surgery. For those who are overweight or have abdominal fat, the risk is further amplified. Individuals with hereditary conditions such as sickle cell disease or hereditary spherocytosis are also at a higher risk, as gallstones can run in families with these conditions.

Symptoms

Many individuals with gallstones experience no symptoms and may not be aware they have them. However, when symptoms do occur, they can be quite distinct. Women over 40 are particularly vulnerable to experiencing biliary colic, a type of abdominal pain that can be severe and persistent, often located in the upper right abdomen. This pain can radiate to the back, right shoulder, or chest and is commonly triggered by fatty meals, usually occurring in the evenings or at night. Biliary colic can sometimes be mistaken for heartburn or indigestion, leading to potential delays in diagnosis.

In addition to biliary colic, other symptoms include cholecystitis, characterized by persistent pain and tenderness in the upper right abdomen, flu-like symptoms, and potential sepsis. Jaundice, a yellowing of the skin and eyes, may occur if a gallstone blocks the bile duct, preventing the removal of bilirubin. This condition can be particularly challenging to detect in individuals with darker skin tones. Cholangitis, a severe infection of the bile ducts caused by a persistent blockage, is a medical emergency and requires immediate attention.

Complications

For women over 40, complications from gallstones can be more severe due to the potential for chronic pain and more pronounced symptoms. If a gallstone obstructs a bile duct, it can lead to intense pain and discomfort, and if the blockage persists, it can result in cholecystitis or cholangitis. These conditions can significantly impact overall health and quality of life. Additionally, rapid weight loss or obesity can exacerbate these complications, as the body's ability to process and manage bile is compromised.

Why a Gallstone Diet is Important for Women Above 40

A tailored gallstone diet is crucial for women over 40 to manage and prevent gallstone-related issues. This diet focuses on reducing cholesterol levels in bile and maintaining a healthy weight, both of which are essential in mitigating the risk of gallstone formation. By incorporating foods that support gallbladder health and avoiding those that can trigger gallstone symptoms, such as high-fat and cholesterol-rich foods, women can better manage their risk and alleviate symptoms. Additionally, this diet helps address weight-related risk factors, supporting overall health and potentially reducing the frequency of gallstone attacks.

The Role of Age and Gender in Fighting Gallstone

Age and gender play significant roles in the development and management of gallstones. For women over 40, hormonal changes, combined with an increased risk of obesity and related health conditions, heighten their susceptibility. Understanding these factors helps in creating effective prevention and management strategies, including a specialized diet and lifestyle adjustments that align with their specific health needs. By addressing these elements proactively, women can better manage their gallstone risk and maintain overall health.

CHAPTER II

HORMONAL CHANGES AND GALLSTONE FORMATION

For women over 40, hormonal changes significantly impact gallstone formation. Estrogen, the primary female sex hormone, plays a crucial role in regulating various bodily functions, including the menstrual cycle and the thickening of the uterine lining. However, estrogen is also linked to gallstone formation. This hormone can affect the composition of bile and the function of the gallbladder, increasing the likelihood of gallstones. Women in their forties often experience hormonal fluctuations that can exacerbate this risk, making gallstone management particularly pertinent for this age group.

The "4F factor"—fertile, fat, flatulent (constipation), and forty—highlights the increased risk for women in this demographic. These factors combine with hormonal changes to heighten the probability of gallstone formation. Estrogen dominance, in particular, plays a significant role. This condition occurs when estrogen levels are disproportionately high relative to progesterone. Estrogen dominance can cause the Sphincter of Oddi, the muscle controlling bile flow into the duodenum, to constrict. This constriction hampers bile flow, leading to the formation of biliary sludge, which can solidify into gallstones over time.

Hormonal Health and Gallstones

Maintaining hormonal health is crucial for women over 40 to mitigate the risk of gallstones. The intricate balance of hormones like estrogen and progesterone influences various physiological processes, including bile production and gallbladder function. Estrogen dominance, whether due to natural hormonal changes, infertility treatments, or hormone replacement therapy (HRT), increases the risk of gallstones. Understanding this connection allows for more proactive management of gallstone risks through diet, lifestyle changes, and medical interventions when necessary.

For women undergoing infertility treatments or estrogen therapy, the risk of gallstone formation is particularly high. These treatments often involve high doses of estrogen, exacerbating the likelihood of bile sludge and gallstone formation. Monitoring hormonal health and seeking medical advice can help manage these risks effectively.

Impact of Menopause

Menopause marks a significant hormonal shift for women, typically occurring in their late 40s or early 50s. This transition can significantly impact gallstone risk due to changes in estrogen and progesterone levels. During menopause, estrogen levels decline, but periods of estrogen dominance can still occur, particularly with HRT. These fluctuations can disrupt bile composition and gallbladder function, increasing the risk of gallstones.

Postmenopausal women often experience changes in body weight and fat distribution, which further contribute to gallstone risk. Abdominal fat, in particular, is linked to higher cholesterol levels in bile, a key factor in gallstone formation. Therefore, managing weight and maintaining a balanced diet are essential strategies for mitigating gallstone risk during and after menopause.

Hormone Replacement Therapy (HRT)

Hormone Replacement Therapy (HRT) is commonly used to alleviate menopausal symptoms, but it also carries an increased risk of gallstones. Over 6.3 million females in the United States between the ages of 20 and 74 have gallstones, with prevalence increasing with age. HRT often involves supplemental estrogen, which can lead to estrogen dominance. This condition exacerbates the risk of gallstones by affecting bile composition and flow.

Estrogen therapy, whether for menopausal symptoms or infertility treatments, can increase the likelihood of biliary sludge and gallstone formation. Women on HRT should be aware of these risks and work with healthcare providers to monitor and manage their hormone levels effectively. Dietary adjustments, such as increasing fiber intake and maintaining a healthy weight, can also help mitigate the risk.

CHAPTER III

THE BASICS OF A GALLSTONE DIET

Gallstones are small, hard deposits that form in the gallbladder. They can cause significant discomfort and health issues, particularly for women over 40, who are more prone to developing them due to hormonal changes. A specialized diet can help manage and reduce the risk of gallstones by promoting healthy digestion and preventing the formation of these stones.

Principles of a Gallstone Diet

A gallstone diet focuses on several key principles:

- Low Fat Intake: Consuming low-fat foods helps reduce the cholesterol levels in bile, which is a primary component in gallstone formation.

- High Fiber: Fiber aids in digestion and can help prevent the formation of cholesterol gallstones.

- Hydration: Staying well-hydrated ensures that bile can flow easily and prevents the formation of gallstones.

- Regular Meals: Eating regular, balanced meals prevents the gallbladder from becoming overworked and helps maintain a steady bile flow.

Foods to Avoid

Certain foods can increase the risk of gallstone formation or exacerbate symptoms if you already have gallstones. These include:

- High-Fat Foods: Avoid foods high in saturated fats such as butter, cream, fatty cuts of meat, and full-fat dairy products.
- Fried Foods: These are often high in unhealthy fats that can contribute to gallstone formation.
- Sugary Foods: Limit the intake of sweets, pastries, and sugary beverages.
- Refined Carbohydrates: Avoid white bread, pasta, and other refined grains that lack fiber.

Foods to Include

Incorporating the right foods into your diet can help manage and prevent gallstones:

- Fruits and Vegetables: Aim for a variety of colors and types to get a wide range of nutrients and antioxidants.
- Whole Grains: Include 100% whole grains like oats, quinoa, brown rice, and whole wheat products.
- Lean Proteins: Opt for lean cuts of meat, poultry, fish, and plant-based proteins like beans and legumes.
- Healthy Fats: Use small amounts of healthy fats from sources like avocados, nuts, seeds, and olive oil.

Creating a Gallstone-Friendly Meal Plan

A gallstone-friendly meal plan focuses on balanced, nutrient-dense foods that are low in fat and high in fiber. Here is an example of a day's meals:

Breakfast:

- Oatmeal with fresh berries and a sprinkle of chia seeds.
- A cup of herbal tea or coffee (without cream).

Mid-Morning Snack:

- An apple or a handful of nuts.

Lunch:

- A large salad with mixed greens, cherry tomatoes, cucumbers, chickpeas, and a lemon vinaigrette.
- A serving of whole grain bread.

Afternoon Snack:

- Carrot sticks with hummus.

Dinner:

- Grilled salmon or tofu with steamed broccoli and quinoa.
- A side of mixed vegetables drizzled with a small amount of olive oil.

Evening Snack:

- A bowl of low-fat yogurt with a teaspoon of honey and sliced almonds.

Tips for a Gallstone-Friendly Lifestyle

- Stay Hydrated: Drink plenty of water throughout the day to aid digestion and bile flow.

- Moderate Alcohol: Research indicates that moderate alcohol consumption, such as a glass of wine, may reduce the risk of gallstones.

- Avoid Skipping Meals: Eating at regular intervals helps maintain a steady flow of bile.

- Gradual Weight Loss: If you need to lose weight, aim for a gradual weight loss of 1-2 pounds per week to avoid increasing the risk of gallstones.

- Healthy Cooking Methods: Opt for steaming, baking, grilling, or boiling instead of frying.

By adhering to these guidelines and focusing on a balanced, low-fat, high-fiber diet, women over 40 can significantly reduce their risk of gallstones and manage any existing symptoms more effectively.

CHAPTER IV

BREAKFAST RECIPES FOR GALLSTONE IN WOMEN ABOVE 40

Tofu Scramble Breakfast Tacos

INGREDIENTS

for 1 serving

1 tablespoon olive oil

⅓ block tofu

1 tablespoon low sodium soy sauce

1 tablespoon nutritional yeast

½ teaspoon turmeric

¾ teaspoon garlic powder

black pepper, to taste

1 cup spinach(40 g)

2 whole wheat tortillas

¼ avocado, sliced

½ red pepper, diced

INSTRUCTIONS

In a medium-sized sauté pan, add olive oil and tofu, and sauté until lightly browned.

Add in soy sauce, nutritional yeast, garlic powder, turmeric, black pepper, red pepper, and spinach, then sauté for 3-5 more minutes or until spinach is wilted.

Serve immediately on tortillas and top with avocado, and hot sauce.

Enjoy!

Creamy Strawberry Balsamic Avocado Toast

INGREDIENTS

for 1 serving

bread, toasted

2 tablespoons goat cheese

½ avocado, sliced

4 strawberries, sliced

balsamic vinegar

INSTRUCTIONS

Spread the goat cheese on toast.

Add sliced avocados, strawberries, and drizzle with balsamic vinegar.

Enjoy!

Broccoli Cheddar Brunch Bake

INGREDIENTS

for 4 servings

12 eggs, whisked

salt, to taste

pepper, to taste

½ onion, diced

½ cup shredded cheddar cheese(50 g)

1 cup cherry tomato(200 g), halved

1 head small broccoli floret

scallion, for garnish, optional

INSTRUCTIONS

Preheat oven to 325°F (160°C).

In a large bowl, whisk 12 eggs with salt and pepper.

Add onion and cheese and combine.

In an oiled baking dish, add tomatoes, broccoli, and egg mixture.

Bake for 30-45 minutes or until golden and eggs are set.

Garnish with scallions.

Enjoy!

Nutrient-Packed Colorful Super Salad

INGREDIENTS

for 6 servings

3 tablespoons wole grain mustard

2 tablespoons organic maple syrup

1 tablespoon fresh ginger, grated

4 cloves garlic, grated

1 tablespoon sesame seed, toasted

¼ teaspoon cayenne pepper

¼ cup apple cider vinegar(60 mL)

¼ cup lemon juice(60 mL)

⅓ cup extra virgin olive oil(80 mL)

kosher salt, to taste

black pepper, to taste

2 cups lacinato kale(135 g), thinly sliced

2 large carrots, peeled and grated

2 cups broccoli floret(300 g)

2 cups red cabbage(200 g), thinly sliced

1 red bell pepper, seeded and thinly sliced

1 avocado, peeled and cubed

1 cup walnut(100 g), chopped

½ cup fresh parlsey(20 g), chopped

INSTRUCTIONS

In a liquid measuring cup, combine the mustard, maple syrup, ginger, garlic, sesame seeds, cayenne, apple cider vinegar, lemon juice, and olive oil. Whisk until fully incorporated. Season to taste with salt and pepper.

Add the kale, carrots, red cabbage, broccoli, red cabbage, bell pepper, avocado, walnuts, and parsley to a large serving bowl.

Pour desired amount of dressing over the salad and toss until everything is well coated.

Garnish with more toasted sesame seeds

Finger Sandwiches

INGREDIENTS

for 12 finger sandwiches

CHEESE AND CHUTNEY

2 slices brown bread

1 tablespoon chutney

2 slices cheddar cheese

HAM AND MUSTARD

2 slices white bread

1 tablespoon wholegrain mustard

2 slices ham

SALMON AND CREAM CHEESE

2 slices white bread

1 tablespoon cream cheese

2 slices smoked salmon

fresh dill

CUCUMBER

2 slices granary bread

1 tablespoon butter

¼ cucumber, peeled, cut into slices

salt

pepper

INSTRUCTIONS

While the tortes are chilling, get started on the sandwiches.

Assemble each sandwich and cut off the crusts.

Lay out on a plate and leave to chill in the fridge.

Enjoy!

Lentil Bolognese

INGREDIENTS

for 8 servings

2 medium carrots, roughly chopped

1 large white onion, roughly chopped

3 celeries, roughly chopped

3 cloves garlic

1 cup raw walnut(100 g)

2 tablespoons olive oil

1 teaspoon dried basil

2 teaspoons dried oregano

1 teaspoon dried parsley

kosher salt, to taste

2 tablespoons tomato paste

2 ¾ cups low sodium vegetable broth(660 mL)

1 cup green lentil(200 g)

1 can diced tomato

½ cup red wine(120 mL)

noodle, for serving

6 medium zucchinis

2 tablespoons olive oil, plus more as needed

kosher salt, to taste

½ teaspoon red pepper flakes

3 cloves garlic, minced

6 medium zucchinis

2 tablespoons olive oil, plus more as needed

kosher salt, to taste

½ teaspoon red pepper flakes

3 cloves garlic, minced

INSTRUCTIONS

In a food processor, combine the carrots, onion, celery, and garlic. Pulse until finely chopped, but not mushy. Transfer the vegetables to a bowl.

Add the walnuts to the food processor and pulse until they reach the consistency of ground meat.

Heat the olive oil in a large pot over medium-high heat. Add the vegetable mixture, basil, oregano, parsley, and salt. Cook for 25 minutes, stirring frequently, until caramelized and any excess moisture has evaporated. Add the tomato paste, stir to combine, and cook for 5 minutes.

Add the vegetable stock, lentils, ground walnuts, and tomatoes and season with salt. Reduce the heat to medium, cover, and simmer for 35 minutes, stirring occasionally, until the lentils are cooked through and walnuts have softened. Remove the lid and cook off any remaining liquid, stirring frequently, about 5 minutes.

Add the wine, stir, and reduce until there is no liquid at the bottom of the pot, about 10 minutes. Season with more salt to taste.

Trim the ends of the zucchini, then cut into noodles using a spiralizer or julienne peeler.

Add 2 tablespoons of olive oil, a pinch of salt, the red pepper flakes, and garlic to a large pan. Turn the heat to medium and cook for 2-3 minutes, until the garlic is fragrant.

Work in batches, add about 2-3 cups of zucchini noodles at a time to the pan. Season lightly with salt and cook for 45-60 seconds, tossing continuously with tongs, until warmed through. 9. Add more olive oil, 1 tablespoon at a time, if the pan looks dry.

Serve the zucchini noodles with the Bolognese.

Enjoy!

Spice-Rubbed Flank Steak Salad

INGREDIENTS

for 5 servings

1 lb flank steak(455 g)

salt, to taste

pepper, to taste

1 teaspoon garlic powder, to taste

onion powder, to taste

cayenne pepper, to taste

oil, your preference

5 cups mixed greens(1 kg)

1 cup cherry tomatoes(200 g)

2 avocados, diced

1 cup carrot(110 g), shredded

½ red onion, sliced

HONEY MUSTARD DRESSING

2 tablespoons mustard

2 tablespoons honey

2 tablespoons lemon juice

1 tablespoon olive oil

¼ teaspoon salt

¼ teaspoon pepper

INSTRUCTIONS

Season both sides of the flank steak generously with salt, pepper, garlic powder, onion powder, and cayenne. Massage the spices into the steak well.

In an oiled skillet, cook steak for 2-3 minutes on both sides (depending on desired doneness), flipping once.

Remove steak from skillet and allow to rest on a cutting board for 10 minutes. Allowing the steak to rest before cutting it allows the juices to resettle.

While the steak rests, combine the mustard, honey, lemon juice, olive oil, salt, and pepper in a small bowl. Whisk to combine. Set aside.

Cut the steak against the grain.

Assemble the salad with mixed greens, cherry tomatoes, avocados, shredded carrots, and red onion. Top with cut steak.

Serve with dressing.

Roasted Summer Veggies

INGREDIENTS

for 4 servings

2 zucchinis, skin on, cut into 3/4 inch (2 cm) cubes

2 eggplants, skin on, cut into 3/4 inch (2 cm) cubes

1 yellow onion, thinly sliced

3 cloves garlic, minced

¼ cup extra virgin olive oil(60 mL)

2 teaspoons kosher salt

7 roma tomatoes

INSTRUCTIONS

Preheat the oven at 350°F (180°C).

While it's heating, chop zucchini, eggplant, onion, and garlic.

Then toss them in a large bowl with salt, pepper, and oil. Transfer to a foil-lined sheet tray.

Bake for 40 minutes, stirring every 10 minutes.

Meanwhile, score a small 'X' into the bottom of each tomato and microwave them in a bowl for 7 to 10 minutes.

Once cooled, peel the skin off and roughly dice them.

After 40 minutes of cooking, increase oven to 400°F (205°C), add the tomatoes, and bake for an additional 25 minutes.

Let cool, then store in covered container in fridge.

Sweet Potato "Fried" Rice

INGREDIENTS

for 2 servings

2 medium-sized sweet potatoes, peeled and chopped

1 tablespoon cooking oil, of preference, or water

½ white onion, diced

2 large carrots, peeled and sliced

½ teaspoon salt

½ teaspoon pepper

½ cup vegetable broth(120 mL)

½ cup pea(75 g), cooked

2 eggs, scrambled

2 tablespoons low sodium soy sauce

green onion, chopped, for garnish

INSTRUCTIONS

In a food processor, pulse the sweet potato chunks until they reach your desired "rice" consistency.

In a large skillet over medium heat, heat oil, then add onions and let cook until translucent.

Add sweet potato rice, carrots, salt, pepper, and vegetable broth and cook until the liquid has evaporated and the sweet potato is tender, stirring occasionally.

Add peas, eggs, and soy sauce, and combine, allowing it to heat through.

Garnish with green onions.

Enjoy!

Cauliflower & Chickpea Burgers

INGREDIENTS

for 4 servings

1 head cauliflower

1 teaspoon salt

15 oz chickpeas(425 g), 1 can, drained, rinsed

1 small onion, finely chopped

1 red bell pepper, finely chopped

1 clove garlic, minced

⅓ cup fresh cilantro(15 g), finely chopped

1 teaspoon turmeric

½ teaspoon cumin

salt, to taste

black pepper, to taste

HUMMUS

1 tomato, sliced

pickle

INSTRUCTIONS

Preheat oven to 350°F (180°C).

Place a towel over a large bowl. Using a box grater, grate the head of cauliflower down to the stem over the bowl. Add the salt to the cauliflower, mix it in, and allow it to sit for 20 minutes. After 20 minutes, use the towel to wring out the excess water from the cauliflower and return it to the bowl.

Add the chickpeas, onion, bell pepper, garlic, cilantro, and spices to the cauliflower. Using a potato masher, mash the ingredients until thoroughly mixed together.

Take a quarter of the mixture and shape it into a patty using your hands. Repeat with the remaining mixture to create four patties.

Take the patties and place them on a parchment paper-lined baking sheet and bake for 20 minutes.

Place patties on buns, and top with hummus, lettuce, tomato, and pickles.

Enjoy!

Citrus And Winter Greens Salad

INGREDIENTS

for 4 servings

1 clove garlic

¼ cup finely chopped fresh parsley(10 g)

¼ cup chopped scallions(25 g)

¼ cup apple cider vinegar(60 mL)

2 tablespoons honey

¼ cup orange juice(60 mL), reserved from supreming oranges, if desired

1 tablespoon dijon mustard

2 tablespoons tahini

kosher salt, to taste

2 tablespoons extra-virgin olive oil

3 cups thinly sliced Tuscan kale(300 g), packed

1 cup thinly sliced red cabbage(100 g)

1 large fuji apple, cored and thinly sliced

1 cup thinly sliced Brussels sprouts(115 g)

3 oranges, supremed

¼ cup toasted pepitas(30 g)

¼ cup pomegranate seeds(20 g)

INSTRUCTIONS

Make the dressing: Add the garlic, parsley, scallions, apple cider vinegar, honey, orange juice, Dijon mustard, tahini, and salt to a blender. Blend until smooth. With the blender running, slowly drizzle in the olive oil until the dressing is easily pourable. Set aside until ready to use.

15 minutes prior to serving the salad, add the kale to a large bowl and season with salt. Gently massage with your hands to break down the tough fibers and reduce bitterness.

Add the red cabbage, apple, Brussels sprouts, orange segments, pepitas, and pomegranate seeds. Toss well to combine. Divide between serving bowls or plates and drizzle with dressing to taste.

Enjoy!

Jacket Potato

INGREDIENTS

for 4 servings

2 russet potatoes

cooking spray

1 teaspoon kosher salt

½ cup milk or stock(120 mL)

cooked bacon

queso

green onion, thinly sliced

INSTRUCTIONS

Preheat oven to 375°F (190°C). Line a baking sheet with parchment paper.

Thoroughly clean and dry potatoes. Slice in half lengthwise. Spray potatoes liberally with cooking spray season with salt. Place potatoes cut side down on prepared baking sheet.

Roast potatoes for 30 minutes or until the skin is crispy and the center is tender. Set aside to cool for 5 minutes.

Spoon the flesh out of the potato leaving a ¼ inch (½ cm) border of potato in the skin. Place flesh in a bowl and set the skin aside.

To the bowl with the scooped out potato, add milk or stock and stir until smooth. Spoon seasoned potato back into the skins.

Top with bacon, drizzle with queso, and garnish with green onion, to taste.

Enjoy!

Chicken Meatball Soup

INGREDIENTS

for 6 servings

CHICKEN MEATBALLS

1 lb ground chicken(455 g)

½ cup panko bread crumbs(25 g)

1 large egg

½ cup grated parmesan cheese(55 g)

2 cloves garlic, minced

¼ cup finely chopped fresh parsley(10 g)

1 teaspoon kosher salt

½ teaspoon black pepper

1 tablespoon olive oil

SOUP

1 tablespoon olive oil

1 cup diced white onion(150 g)

½ cup diced carrots(60 g)

½ cup diced celery(110 g)

2 cloves garlic, minced

8 cups chicken stock(2 L)

1 dried bay leaf

1 cup dried orzo pasta(145 g)

4 cups roughly chopped Swiss chard(400 g)

3 tablespoons grated parmesan cheese

kosher salt, to taste

black pepper, to taste

1 tablespoon lemon juice

INSTRUCTIONS

Make the meatballs: In a medium bowl, combine the ground chicken, bread crumbs, egg, Parmesan, garlic, parsley, salt, and pepper. Mix well, then roll into 1-inch (2 cm) meatballs. You should have 16-18 total.

In a large pot, heat the olive oil over medium heat. Sear the meatballs on all sides until golden brown, 4-5 minutes. Remove from the pot and set aside.

Make the soup: In the same pot, heat the remaining tablespoon of oil. Add the onion, carrot, and celery and cook, stirring occasionally until tender, 3-4 minutes. Add the garlic and cook until fragrant, 1-2 minutes.

Add the chicken stock and bay leaf. Cover and bring to a boil.

Once boiling, add the orzo and meatballs. Cover and simmer for 7-8 minutes, until the orzo is tender.

Add the Swiss chard, cover, and cook for 2-3 minutes, until the chard has wilted.

Add the Parmesan cheese and season to taste with salt and pepper. Add the lemon juice.

Ladle into bowls and serve.

Enjoy!

Slow-Cooker Collard Greens And Ham Hocks

INGREDIENTS

for 12 servings

3 ½ lb collard green(1.5 kg), washed

1 large yellow onion

2 lb ham(910 g)

1 tablespoon brown sugar

½ teaspoon black pepper

2 teaspoons salt

3 tablespoons apple cider vinegar

32 oz chicken broth(945 mL)

INSTRUCTIONS

Remove the stems from the collard greens, then stack the leaves on top of each other and roughly chop.

Add the collard greens to a slow cooker with the onion, ham hocks, brown sugar, pepper, salt, apple cider vinegar, and chicken broth.

Cover and cook on low for 8 hours or high for 4 hours, until the greens are tender.

Remove the ham hocks from the slow cooker. Trim and discard any fat and bones. Roughly chop the meat and return to the greens. Toss to incorporate.

Serve warm.

INSTRUCTIONS

Remove the stems from the collard greens, then stack the leaves on top of each other and roughly chop.

Add the collard greens to a slow cooker with the onion, ham hocks, brown sugar, pepper, salt, apple cider vinegar, and chicken broth.

Cover and cook on low for 8 hours or high for 4 hours, until the greens are tender.

Remove the ham hocks from the slow cooker. Trim and discard any fat and bones. Roughly chop the meat and return to the greens. Toss to incorporate.

Serve warm.

Vegetarian Potstickers

INGREDIENTS

for 6 servings

3 tablespoons neutral oil, plus 2 teaspoons, divided

1 finely diced yellow onion

1 tablespoon minced fresh ginger

1 tablespoon minced garlic

2 cups finely diced mushrooms(150 g)

¼ cup finely diced bell pepper(25 g), finely diced

2 cups shredded cabbage(200 g)

2 cups shredded carrots(220 g)

kosher salt, to taste

freshly ground black pepper, to taste

1 tablespoon chopped fresh cilantro

1 cup finely chopped green onions(150 g)

2 tablespoons soy sauce, plus more for serving

2 teaspoons sesame oil

3 tablespoons cooking sherry

1 teaspoon sugar

wonton wrapper

¼ cup water(60 mL), plus more for sealing dumplings

dipping sauce

INSTRUCTIONS

Heat 3 tablespoons of oil in a deep pan or wok over medium heat. Add the onion, ginger, and garlic and cook until the onion is translucent.

Add the mushrooms and bell peppers to the pan. Cook until the mushrooms are softened.

Add the cabbage, carrots, salt, and pepper. Cook for another 3-4 minutes, until tender, then remove the pan from the heat. Set aside to cool completely.

Once cooled, add the cilantro, green onions, soy sauce, sesame oil, cooking sherry, and sugar. Mix well.

Add a spoonful of the vegetable mixture to the center of a wonton wrapper. Dip your finger in water and run it around the edge of the dough. Fold the dough over the filling, pleating and pressing the edges together to seal.

Heat the remaining 2 teaspoons of oil in a large skillet over medium heat. Arrange the dumplings in the pan. Cook for 3-4 minutes, or until a crust has started to form on the bottoms. Pour the water in the pan and cover with a lid. Steam for 6-8 minutes, then remove from the pan.

Serve with your choice of dipping sauce or soy sauce.

Enjoy!

Cauliflower Steaks

INGREDIENTS

for 4 servings

1 large head cauliflower

4 tablespoons olive oil

2 tablespoons lemon juice

1 teaspoon dried basil

1 teaspoon dried oregano

1 teaspoon fresh thyme

1 teaspoon dried rosemary

1 teaspoon onion powder

2 cloves garlic, minced

salt, to taste

pepper, to taste

INSTRUCTIONS

Preheat the oven to 400°F (200°C). Line a baking sheet with parchment paper.

Remove the green leaves from the cauliflower stem with a knife.

Place the cauliflower core-down on a cutting board and trim 2 sides so they become flat.

Cut the cauliflower in half and then cut each half in two to get 4 "steaks".

Rinse and dry the cauliflower steaks.

In a small bowl, combine the olive oil, lemon juice, basil, oregano, thyme, rosemary, onion, and garlic, plus salt and pepper to taste. Mix well.

Place the cauliflower steaks on the baking sheet and brush generously with the oil mixture.

Bake for about 25 minutes, flipping halfway, until tender.

Serve as desired, such as on a sandwich with pesto and red pepper, or with barbecue sauce and roasted potatoes, or with vegan mushroom gravy and lentils.

Enjoy!

Focaccia

INGREDIENTS

for 12 servings

⅔ cup warm water(160 mL)

1 tablespoon active dry yeast

1 tablespoon honey

2 ½ cups bread flour(310 g), divided

1 ¾ cups room temperature water

9 tablespoons olive oil, divided, plus more to taste

3 cups all purpose flour(375 g), plus more for dusting

1 tablespoon kosher salt

TOPPINGS

3 sprigs fresh dill

3 sprigs fresh rosemary

2 edible flowers

5 spears asparagus, woody ends trimmed and shaved

4 white mushrooms, cut into 1/3 in (8 mm) slices

3 cherry tomatoes, of varying colors, halved

2 tablespoons kalamata olive, halved

1 tablespoon fresno chilie, thinly sliced

1 watermelon radish, thinly sliced

6 fresh chives

1 radish, thinly sliced

flaky sea salt, to taste

INSTRUCTIONS

In a large bowl, whisk together the warm water, yeast, honey, and ½ cup (60 G) bread flour. Cover the bowl with plastic wrap and set in a warm place for 20–30 minutes, until the mixture is bubbly.

Add the room temperature water, 5 tablespoons of olive oil, remaining 2 cups of bread flour, the all-purpose flour, and salt. Mix well with a rubber spatula to combine until the dough starts to come together.

Turn the dough out onto a surface lightly dusted with all-purpose flour and bring together. Knead for 10–15 minutes, adding flour as needed to prevent sticking. The dough should be smooth and supple and bounce back when pressed.

Coat a large bowl with 1 tablespoon of olive oil and transfer the dough into the bowl. Cover with plastic wrap and let rest in a warm place for 1–2 hours, until doubled in size.

Remove the plastic wrap and punch the dough down.

Grease a 18 x 13-inch (45 x 33 cm) baking sheet with 1-2 tablespoons of olive oil and use your hands to spread the oil all around the pan to coat. Transfer the dough to the pan and cover the dough with the same piece of plastic wrap. Let rest for 10–20 minutes so it is easier to stretch.

Uncover the dough. With oiled hands, gently stretch the dough to fit the size of the baking sheet. Cover with plastic wrap again and let proof at room temperature for 1–2 hours, until the dough rises to fill the pan, or refrigerate overnight. Refrigerating overnight is optional, however it will result in a better final texture and flavor. If refrigerating, let the dough come to room temperature for 30–60 minutes before proceeding, until slightly puffed.

Preheat the oven to 400°F (200°C).

Use your fingers to dimple the surface of the focaccia dough. Drizzle with the remaining 2 tablespoons of olive oil.

Use the dill, rosemary, edible flowers, asparagus, mushrooms, cherry tomatoes, Kalamata olives, Fresno chiles, watermelon radish, chives, and radish to create a decorative gardenscape scene on the focaccia. Sprinkle all over with flaky sea salt.

Bake the focaccia for 15 minutes, then turn the pan and bake for another 7–10 minutes, until the bread is golden brown in the areas not covered with toppings. If the toppings are getting too dark, lightly cover the focaccia with foil for the remainder of baking.

Remove the focaccia from the oven and let cool in the pan for 10 minutes. Transfer to a cutting board and drizzle with more olive oil.

Slice and serve.

CHAPTER V

LUNCH RECIPES FOR GALLSTONE IN WOMEN ABOVE 40

Bibimbap Casserole with Tofu

INGREDIENTS

2 tablespoon gochujang (Korean hot pepper paste)

2 tablespoon soy sauce

1 tablespoon toasted sesame oil

1 tablespoon honey

1 teaspoon rice vinegar

2 tablespoon vegetable oil

1 8 ounce pkg. fresh cremini mushrooms, sliced (3 cups)

1 ½ cup chopped onion

4 cloves garlic, minced

4 cup chopped, stemmed fresh kale

2 cup coarsely shredded carrots

3 cup cooked rice

1 14 ounce pkg. extra-firm tofu, drained and cut into 1-inch cubes

8 eggs

¼ teaspoon salt

¼ teaspoon coarsely ground black pepper

½ cup bias-sliced green onions

2 teaspoon sesame seeds

Sriracha sauce

INSTRUCTIONS

Preheat oven to 450°F. In a small bowl stir together the first five ingredients (through vinegar). In an extra-large skillet heat vegetable oil over medium-high. Add mushrooms, onion, and garlic; cook and stir 5 to 6 minutes or until mushrooms brown. Add kale and carrots; cook and stir 2 minutes more. Add rice and gochujang mixture. Stir to coat. Gently stir in the tofu.

Spoon tofu mixture into a 3-qt. rectangular baking dish, spreading evenly. Make eight indents in the mixture with the back of a spoon. Crack an egg into each indent. Sprinkle with salt and pepper. Cover with foil.

Bake about 20 minutes or until heated through and eggs are just set. Loosen foil. Let stand 10 minutes. Sprinkle with green onions and sesame seeds; serve with sriracha sauce for drizzling.

Celery and Apple Salad with Walnuts

INGREDIENTS

3 tablespoon olive oil

2 tablespoon fresh lemon juice

2 teaspoon honey

1 ½ teaspoon chopped fresh thyme

Salt and black pepper

3 celery stalks with leaves, thinly bias-sliced (1 1/2 cups)

1 medium red apple, cored and thinly sliced

¼ cup thinly sliced red onion

¼ cup coarsely chopped walnuts, toasted

INSTRUCTIONS

In a medium bowl whisk together olive oil, lemon juice, honey, thyme, and salt and pepper to taste.

Add celery, apple, onion, and walnuts; toss to coat.

Salmon with Roasted Tomatoes and Shallots

INGREDIENTS

1 1 pound fresh or frozen salmon fillet, skinned if desired

⅛ teaspoon salt

⅛ teaspoon black pepper

Nonstick cooking spray

4 cup grape and/or cherry tomatoes

½ cup thinly sliced shallots

6 cloves garlic, minced

2 tablespoon chopped fresh oregano or 1 1/2 tsp. dried oregano, crushed

1 tablespoon olive oil

¼ teaspoon salt

¼ teaspoon black pepper

INSTRUCTIONS

Thaw salmon, if frozen. Preheat oven to 400°F. Sprinkle salmon with the 1/8 tsp. each salt and pepper.

Lightly coat a 3-qt. rectangular baking dish with cooking spray. In the baking dish combine the remaining ingredients. Toss to coat.

Roast tomato mixture, uncovered, 15 minutes. Place salmon, skin side down, on top of tomato mixture. Roast, uncovered, 15 to 18 minutes or until salmon flakes easily.

Using two large pancake turners, transfer the salmon to a platter. Top with tomato mixture.

Black Bean-Mango Salsa

INGREDIENTS

2 mangoes, seeded, peeled, and chopped

1 15 ounce can black beans, drained and rinsed

½ cup finely chopped red onion

¼ cup lime juice

2 tablespoon honey

1 tablespoon chopped fresh cilantro

½ teaspoon salt

¼ teaspoon black pepper

INSTRUCTIONS

In a medium bowl mash 1 cup of the chopped mangoes. Stir in remaining chopped mangoes and remaining ingredients. Serve with tortilla chips, grilled meat or poultry, or tacos.

Spicy Green Beans with Herb Salad

INGREDIENTS

2 tablespoon olive oil, plus more for drizzling

4 small shallots, cut into 1/2-inch wedges

4 garlic cloves, thinly sliced

Kosher salt

Freshly ground black pepper

2 - 4 anchovy fillets or 2 tsp. anchovy paste (optional)

¼ - ½ teaspoon crushed red pepper

2 tablespoon apple cider vinegar or white wine vinegar, plus more to finish

1 ½ pound green beans, trimmed

1 cup fresh Italian parsley (leaves and tender stems)

½ cup fresh dill leaves

½ cup fresh mint and/or cilantro (leaves and tender stems)

INSTRUCTIONS

In a large Dutch oven heat the 2 tablespoons oil over medium-high. Add shallots and garlic. Season with salt and black pepper. Cook, without stirring, 4 to 5 minutes or until golden brown on one side. Stir and let them brown a bit more, another 4 to 5 minutes. If desired, add anchovies and let them sizzle and dissolve. Stir in crushed red pepper.

Add the 2 tablespoons vinegar; simmer 1 to 2 minutes. Stir in green beans and 1/2 cup water. Season with salt and black pepper. Simmer, covered, 10 to 12 minutes or until totally tender. Remove from heat. Season with salt, black pepper, and, if desired, additional crushed red pepper.

For herb salad: Toss parsley, dill, and mint with a splash of vinegar and a drizzle of olive oil; season with salt and black pepper.

Transfer bean mixture to a large shallow bowl. Scatter herb salad over beans before serving. Serves 6.

Lemon and Garlic Squid with Samphire, Mango and Pea Salad

INGREDIENTS

400g peas

½ small red onion

200g mango

1 tbsp olive oil

4 medium squid, strips

30g olive spread

100g samphire

90g watercress

50g parsley

1 clove of garlic

Juice of 1 lemon

INSTRUCTIONS

Bring a pan of water to the boil, add the peas and boil for 5 minutes until tender.

Put the chopped onion into a bowl with 1 tbsp of the lemon juice, garlic, olive oil, squid and seasoning then toss together.

Place a frying pan on the heat and pour in the dressed squid and cook until the squid turns opaque. Add the olive spread, samphire and peas then toss together and remove from the heat.

Place the squid, peas and samphire on a serving plate with the watercress and diced mango. Add the rest of the lemon juice before serving.

Mackerel with Red Pepper Quinoa Salad

INGREDIENTS

4 fresh mackerel fillets

200g quinoa

1.5 litres of good quality low-salt vegetable stock

80g rocket

2 cloves of garlic

1 red chilli

170g sugar snap peas or mangetout

250g red pepper, roasted (and rinsed if from a jar)

1 tbsp olive oil

1 small red onion

To serve, young salad leaves

INSTRUCTIONS

For the quinoa salad, put the quinoa into a saucepan with 400ml of the vegetable stock. Bring to the boil and then let simmer for 10 minutes before removing from the heat. Allow the quinoa to absorb any remaining stock.

Meanwhile, add the rocket, garlic, chilli and 100ml of the vegetable stock to a food processor and blend until smooth.

Bring the remaining stock to the boil, add the sugar snap peas/mangetout and boil for 3-5 minutes.

For the mackerel, heat the olive oil in a frying pan. Add the mackerel and fry for 2 minutes on each side and then remove from the pan.

Once the peas/mange tout are cooked, add them to the quinoa, diced red onion, rocket mixture and roasted red peppers. Mix well and serve with the mackerel. Scatter over the young salad leaves if using

Masala Omelette

INGREDIENTS

2 eggs, lightly beaten

1 tbsp finely chopped onion

½ red pepper, seeds removed, chopped

1 tbsp chopped fresh coriander

1 green chilli finely chopped (or to taste)

1 chopped tomato

1 tsp rapeseed oil

INSTRUCTIONS

Combine all the ingredients (except the oil) in a bowl and mix well.

Put the oil in a non- stick frying pan over a medium-hot heat. When hot, pour in the egg mixture.

Keep mixing the egg whilst it is solidifying, when semi-solid let it form into an omelette shape

Turn the omelette over and press down.

Remove when cooked through and serve immediately.

Mushroom and Lentil Soup

INGREDIENTS

1 tablespoon olive oil

2 small onions, roughly chopped

2 sticks celery, roughly chopped

1 carrot, roughly chopped

400g mushrooms, roughly sliced

100g green lentils, pre-cooked in boiling water

1 litre vegetable stock, made from 2 low-salt vegetable stock cubes

1 bay leaf

1 tbsp Worcester sauce

Ground black pepper

Optional to serve - 4 tsp toasted pine nuts

Optional to serve - 4 tsp soya yogurt

INSTRUCTIONS

Sweat the onions in the olive oil for a few minutes until softened, taking care not to colour them.

Add the celery and carrot and continue to stir and cook for a few minutes on a low heat

Set aside a few slices of mushrooms as a garnish, then add the remaining mushrooms, cooked lentils, vegetable stock, Worcester Sauce and bay leaf to the pan and simmer until all the vegetables are cooked and tender

Remove the bay leaf and using a hand blender puree the soup

Season with black pepper and serve, garnished with reserved sliced mushrooms, pine nuts and yogurt, if using.

CHAPTER VI

DINNER RECIPES FOR GALLSTONE IN WOMEN ABOVE 40

Traditional Spanish Paella

INGREDIENTS

1 tbsp olive oil

2 chicken breasts cut into chunks

50g king prawns

100g mussels

1 clove of garlic

3 medium tomatoes, chopped

200g paella rice

Pinch of saffron

1L low salt chicken stock

100g cherry tomatoes

100g broad beans

INSTRUCTIONS

In a large pan, heat the olive oil and fry the chicken for 2 minutes. Add the prawns, mussels, garlic and tomatoes and fry for 2 more minutes.

Sprinkle in the rice and shake the pan. Add the saffron and pour in the boiling chicken stock.

Add the chopped tomatoes and broad beans, season and then let simmer for 20 minutes.

You may need to add more fluid if the rice appears to be drying out

Check the seasoning before serving.

Chickpea Pasta with Mushrooms & Kale

INGREDIENTS

8 ounces chickpea rotini or penne (see Tip)

¼ cup extra-virgin olive oil

2 large cloves garlic, sliced

Pinch of crushed red pepper

8 cups chopped kale

8 ounces cremini mushrooms, quartered

½ teaspoon dried thyme

½ teaspoon salt

Grated Parmesan cheese for serving (optional)

INSTRUCTIONS

Cook pasta according to package directions. Reserve 1 cup of the cooking water, then drain.

Meanwhile, heat oil in a large skillet over medium heat. Add garlic and crushed red pepper; cook, stirring once, until fragrant, about 1 minute. Add kale, mushrooms, thyme and salt; cook, stirring occasionally, until the vegetables are soft, about 5 minutes.

Stir in the pasta and enough of the reserved water to coat; cook, stirring, until combined and hot, about 1 minute more. Serve topped with Parmesan, if desired.

Tip:

We chose chickpea pasta for this dish instead of whole-wheat because it's packed with tons of fiber, protein and nutrients—some brands provide more than 40% of your daily recommended fiber, plus 20 grams of protein per serving. Look for it with other gluten-free pastas.

Winter Vegetable Mulligatawny Soup

INGREDIENTS

3 tablespoons extra-virgin olive oil, divided

1 medium onion, finely chopped

2 medium carrots, finely chopped

1 medium parsnip, peeled and finely chopped

4 cups peeled diced acorn squash or butternut squash

1 medium green apple, peeled and finely chopped

1 tablespoon curry powder

3 cloves garlic, minced, divided

1 teaspoon grated fresh ginger

4 cups low-sodium vegetable broth

1 (14 ounce) can no-salt-added diced tomatoes

½ cup red lentils, picked over and rinsed

2 whole-wheat naan flatbreads, halved

¼ cup chopped fresh cilantro, plus more for garnish

INSTRUCTIONS

Preheat oven to 375°F. Line a baking sheet with foil.

Heat 2 tablespoons oil in a large saucepan over medium heat until shimmering. Add onion, carrots and parsnip and cook until the onions are translucent, about 6 minutes. Add squash, apple, curry powder, 2 cloves garlic and ginger and cook, stirring, until fragrant, 1 to 2 minutes. Add broth, tomatoes and lentils and stir to combine. Bring to a boil. Reduce heat to maintain a low simmer, cover and cook until the squash and lentils are tender, about 20 minutes.

Meanwhile, brush one side of each naan with the remaining 1 tablespoon oil. Sprinkle with the remaining 1 clove garlic and place on the prepared baking sheet. Bake until warmed, 5 to 6 minutes. Remove from oven and sprinkle with cilantro.

Gently mash some of the soup with a potato masher to achieve desired consistency. (Alternatively, transfer half the soup to a blender and puree. Use caution when blending hot liquids.) Garnish the soup with cilantro and serve with the naan.

To make ahead

Refrigerate for up to 4 days.

Savory Sweet potato curry

INGREDIENTS

1 medium size sweet potato, peeled and cut into 2cm pieces

2 tbsp rapeseed or sunflower oil

2 medium size onions, finely diced

3 garlic cloves, peeled and crushed

10g fresh root ginger, peeled and finely grated

1 tsp sweet paprika

2 tsps ground tumeric

1 tsp medium curry powder

¼ tsp hot chilli powder

1 tsp ground coriander

1 tsp garam masala

4 green cardamom pods, crushed

227g can chopped tomatoes

1 tbsp tomato purée

½ green pepper, deseeded and cut into 1cm pieces

1 green chilli, finely diced

250ml reduced salt vegetable stock

2 medium tomatoes, quartered

A small pinch salt

400g can chickpeas, drained and rinsed

For the garam masala 'raita'

150g pot Alpro Plain No Sugars alternative to yogurt

1 tsp garam masala

½ tbsp dried mint

INSTRUCTIONS

Preheat the oven to 190°C/170°C Fan/Gas mark 5.

Line a baking tray with baking parchment. Toss the sweet potato pieces with 1 tablespoon oil and spread out on the tray. Bake for 20-25 minutes until lightly caramelised and tender.

Meanwhile, add the remaining 1 tablespoon oil to a medium saucepan and warm over a low to medium heat. Fry the onions for 8-10 minutes, or until very soft. Add the crushed garlic and ginger and stirring cook for another 1-2 minutes.

Stir in the paprika, turmeric, curry powder, chilli powder, coriander, garam masala and crushed cardamom pods to make a thick paste. Cook for 1-2 minutes, adding a little extra oil if it seems dry.

Add the canned tomatoes and tomato purée and cook for 2-3 minutes until it becomes a paste again. Add the green pepper, green chilli, vegetable stock, fresh tomatoes and a pinch of salt. Bring to a simmer then reduce the heat to low and cook gently for 35-45 minutes until the sauce has thickened. Add the chickpeas and sweet potato to the curry and warm through.

To make the garam masala 'raita', mix all the ingredients together and season. Serve with the curry.

Scrumptious vegetable curry

INGREDIENTS

150g frozen diced butternut squash

½ Aubergine, diced

3 squirts of spray oil

1 tbsp vegetable oil

1 medium onion, chopped

1 clove garlic, finely chopped

1 x 5cm fresh ginger, peeled and finely chopped

1 x red chilli, deseeded and finely sliced

1 tsp ground turmeric

1 tsp ground coriander

1 tsp ground cumin

1 tbsp Garam Masala

100g mushrooms, sliced

1 medium sized courgette, sliced

1 red pepper, chopped

200g passata

300ml reduced salt vegetable stock

6 cherry tomatoes, cut in half

2 x 400g tinned chickpeas, drained

1 tsp vegetable oil

1 tsp coriander seeds

1 tsp cumin seeds

1 tsp onion seeds

150ml soya coconut yoghurt

Handful fresh coriander, chopped

INSTRUCTIONS

Preheat the oven to 190C/ 170C Fan/ Gas Mark 5. Place the diced butternut squash and aubergine onto a baking sheet. Spray with the 3 squirts of oil and mix thoroughly. Cook in the oven for 20 minutes.

Meanwhile, heat the oil in a large frying pan and add the chopped onion. Cook on a gentle heat for 5 minutes or until the onion has softened. Add the garlic, ginger and chilli and cook for a further minute. Stir in the spices and cook for around 30 seconds or until the spices release their fragrance. Add the mushrooms, courgette and pepper into the pan and cook for a few minutes until they start to soften. Pour in the stock, passata and cherry tomatoes and give everything a good stir. Simmer for 15 minutes, stirring occasionally to stop the mixture from sticking to the bottom of the pan.

After 15 minutes add the chickpeas, roasted butternut squash and aubergine to the mixture. Stir through and cook gently for a further 15 minutes, or until the sauce has thickened. Continue to stir occasionally.

In a separate small frying pan, heat 1 teaspoon of oil. When hot, add the cumin seeds, coriander seeds and onion seeds. Fry for a couple of minutes, or until the seeds start to sizzle. Remove from the heat.

Once the curry has thickened, remove from the heat and stir through the yoghurt, fried seeds and fresh coriander. Serve with rice.

Cauliflower "Rice" Tabbouleh

INGREDIENTS

5 tablespoons extra-virgin olive oil, divided

2 ½ teaspoons ground cumin, divided

1 ½ teaspoons dried marjoram

¾ teaspoon salt, divided

¼ teaspoon ground allspice

¼ teaspoon cayenne pepper

1 pound boneless, skinless chicken breast, trimmed

¼ cup lemon juice

2 cups fresh riced cauliflower (see Tip)

2 cups flat-leaf parsley leaves

1 cup diced cucumber

1 cup halved cherry tomatoes

¼ cup sliced scallions

INSTRUCTIONS

Preheat grill to medium-high.

Mix 2 tablespoons oil, 2 teaspoons cumin, marjoram, 1/2 teaspoon salt, allspice and cayenne in a small bowl. Brush on chicken.

Grill the chicken, turning occasionally, until an instant-read thermometer inserted in the thickest part registers 165 degrees F, 10 to 12 minutes.

Meanwhile, whisk lemon juice with the remaining 3 tablespoons oil, 1/2 teaspoon cumin and 1/4 teaspoon salt in a large bowl. Add riced cauliflower, parsley, cucumber, tomatoes and scallions; toss to coat.

Transfer the chicken to a clean cutting board and let rest for 5 minutes. Thinly slice the chicken and serve over the tabbouleh.

Savory Veggie Stew

INGREDIENTS

900g root vegetables: a combination of potatoes, pumpkin/squash and sweet potato

2 onions

½ red chilli pepper (optional)

4cm ginger, grated

2 garlic cloves, crushed

2 tbsp olive oil

1½ tbsp garam masala or ras el hanout

1 tbsp curry powder

1 tsp turmeric

500ml tomato passata

600ml water

Bunch fresh coriander, chopped

200g spinach

220g Alpro Greek Style Plain alternative to yogurt

A pinch of salt and pepper

1 lime, juice

INSTRUCTIONS

Peel the root vegetables, remove the pips from the pumpkin/squash and cut into equal sized chunks. Finely chop the onions and red chilli if using.

Heat the oil in a large pan and over a medium heat fry the chopped onions for about 5-8 minutes until translucent. Add the crushed garlic, grated ginger and chopped chilli and cook for another 1-2 minutes stirring. Add the garam masala or ras el hanout, curry powder and turmeric and cook for 1-2 minutes, stirring to release all the wonderful aromas.

Add the chopped root vegetables, tomato passata, water and chopped coriander. Stir everything together, bring to a simmer and on low heat, simmer for 20-30 minutes until the root vegetables are soft but still maintain their shape.

Add the spinach and Alpro Plain Greek Style and simmer for a further 2 minutes just to wilt the spinach.

Season with a small pinch of salt and a little lime juice.

Salmon & Avocado Salad

INGREDIENTS

½ cup loosely packed fresh dill, plus more for garnish

2 tablespoons water

2 tablespoons lemon juice

2 tablespoons white-wine vinegar

1 teaspoon Dijon mustard

1 small clove garlic

2 avocados, chopped, divided

¼ cup extra-virgin olive oil, plus 1 teaspoon, divided

½ teaspoon salt, divided

4 (5 ounce) skinless salmon fillets

¼ teaspoon ground pepper

3 cups spring mix salad greens

2 cups thinly sliced red cabbage

1 cup matchstick carrots

INSTRUCTIONS

Place dill, water, lemon juice, vinegar, mustard, garlic, 1/2 cup avocado, 1/4 cup oil and 1/4 teaspoon salt in a blender. Process until smooth, about 30 seconds. Refrigerate until ready to use.

Heat the remaining 1 teaspoon oil in a large cast-iron skillet over medium-high heat. Sprinkle salmon evenly with pepper and the remaining 1/4 teaspoon salt. Add the salmon to the pan; cook until golden on the bottom and mostly opaque around the sides, about 4 minutes. Carefully flip the fillets; remove from heat. Let the fillets stand in the pan until cooked through, 2 to 3 minutes.

Combine salad greens, cabbage, carrots and the reserved dressing in a large bowl; toss gently until evenly coated. Divide the salad among 4 plates; top with the remaining avocado. Top each salad with a salmon fillet; garnish with additional dill, if desired.

Cauliflower Fajita Skillet

INGREDIENTS

1 medium head cauliflower, trimmed and thinly sliced

1 medium red bell pepper, sliced

1 medium onion, sliced

3 tablespoons extra-virgin olive oil

1 ½ teaspoons chili powder

1 teaspoon ground cumin

½ teaspoon ground coriander

½ teaspoon salt

¼ teaspoon ground pepper

½ cup pico de gallo

¼ cup chopped pickled jalapeño peppers

Chopped fresh cilantro for garnish

1 14-ounce can light-in-sodium refried beans, warmed

12 corn tortillas, warmed

INSTRUCTIONS

Position a rack in top third of oven and place a large cast-iron skillet on it. Preheat to 425°F.

Combine cauliflower, bell pepper, onion and oil in a medium bowl and toss to coat. Sprinkle with chili powder, cumin, coriander, salt and pepper and toss until well coated. Carefully add the mixture to the hot pan. Roast, stirring once, until the vegetables are tender, about 30 minutes.

Set broiler to high. Broil the vegetables until lightly browned, about 2 minutes.

Top the vegetables with pico de gallo, jalapeños and cilantro, if desired. Serve with refried beans and tortillas.

Grilled Red Snapper

INGREDIENTS

¼ cup mayonnaise

2 tablespoons chopped pickled jalapeños

2 teaspoons whole-grain mustard

1 teaspoon grated lime zest

1 teaspoon lime juice

4 ½ teaspoons chili powder, divided

1 teaspoon ground coriander

¼ teaspoon salt, divided

¼ teaspoon ground pepper

1 ¼ pounds red snapper fillet, cut into 4 portions and patted dry

Cooking spray

1 pound okra

1 tablespoon canola oil

INSTRUCTIONS

Preheat grill to medium-high.

Combine mayonnaise, jalapeños, mustard and lime juice in a small bowl and set aside.

Combine lime zest, 4 teaspoons chili powder, coriander, 1/8 teaspoon salt and pepper in a shallow bowl. Dredge fish with the spice mixture and coat with cooking spray. Toss okra with oil and the remaining 1/2 teaspoon chili powder and 1/8 teaspoon salt. Thread the okra crosswise onto four 12-inch bamboo or metal skewers.

Oil the grill rack. Grill the okra, flipping once halfway, until softened and charred in spots, 4 to 6 minutes. Grill the fish, flipping once halfway, until the flesh is opaque, 4 to 5 minutes. Serve with the reserved sauce.

Mediterranean Vegetable Lasagne

INGREDIENTS

2 aubergines, cut into chunks

2 red onions, cut into wedges

2 red peppers, cut into strips

4 garlic cloves, finely chopped

3 tablespoons olive oil

450g courgettes, sliced

225g lasagne sheets

30g parmesan cheese

For the sauce:

900ml skimmed milk

60g olive spread

70g plain flour

125g reduced fat hard cheese (we used Edam)

INSTRUCTIONS

Preheat the oven to 220°C/fan200°C/gas 7. Mix the aubergine, onion, pepper, garlic and half the oil in a bowl. Transfer to a large roasting tin and cook for 30 minutes or until soft.

Meanwhile, heat the rest of the oil in a frying pan. Fry the courgettes for 4 minutes until browned.

Remove the roasted veg from the oven and stir in the courgettes. Lower the oven to 200°C/fan180°C/gas 6.

For the sauce, bring the milk to the boil in a pan and set aside. Melt the olive spread in a pan, add the flour and cook for 1 minute then remove from the heat. Gradually stir in the milk then bring to the boil whilst stirring and then simmer gently for 10 minutes stirring occasionally.

Cook the lasagne according to the packet instructions.

Add the cheese to the sauce and season with pepper. Spoon a thin layer over the base of a lightly-oiled ovenproof dish, cover with 4 lasagne sheets, overlapping them slightly. Top with half the vegetables, then one-third of the remaining sauce and another 4 sheets of lasagne. Repeat this process once more and then spread over the remaining sauce and sprinkle with Parmesan. Bake for 40 minutes, until golden.

Chopped Salad with Shrimp, Apples & Pecans

INGREDIENTS

5 tablespoons reduced-fat sour cream or plain Greek yogurt

3 tablespoons extra-virgin olive oil

3 tablespoons cider vinegar

¼ cup chopped fresh cilantro

1 tablespoon finely chopped shallot

1 clove garlic, minced

¾ teaspoon dry mustard

¼ teaspoon salt

¼ teaspoon ground pepper

5 cups chopped romaine lettuce

1 pound cooked shrimp, chopped

1 medium red apple, chopped

1 cup chopped radicchio

1 cup chopped celery

½ cup toasted chopped pecans

½ cup shredded carrot

INSTRUCTIONS

Whisk sour cream (or yogurt), oil, vinegar, cilantro, shallot, garlic, mustard, salt and pepper in a large bowl. Add romaine, shrimp, apple, radicchio, celery, pecans and carrots; toss to coat.

CHAPTER VII

DESSERT RECIPES FOR GALLSTONE IN WOMEN ABOVE 40

Apple Pie Filling

INGREDIENTS

18 cups thinly sliced apples

3 tablespoons lemon juice

10 cups water

4 ½ cups white sugar

1 cup cornstarch

2 teaspoons ground cinnamon

1 teaspoon salt

¼ teaspoon ground nutmeg

INSTRUCTIONS

Place apples in a bowl. Toss apples with lemon juice in a large bowl and set aside.

Pour water into a Dutch oven over medium heat. Combine sugar, cornstarch, cinnamon, salt, and nutmeg in a bowl; add to water, stir well, and bring to a boil. Boil for 2 minutes, constantly stirring.

Add apples and return to a boil. Reduce heat, cover, and simmer until apples are tender, 6 to 8 minutes. Cool for 30 minutes.

Ladle into 5 freezer containers, leaving 1/2 inch of headspace. Cool at room temperature no longer than 1 1/2 hours.

Seal and freeze. Can be stored for up to 12 months.

Enjoy!

Canned Apple Pie Filling

INGREDIENTS

4 ½ cups white sugar

1 cup cornstarch

2 teaspoons ground cinnamon

¼ teaspoon ground nutmeg

10 cups water

2 teaspoons salt

3 tablespoons lemon juice

2 drops yellow food coloring (Optional)

6 pounds apples

INSTRUCTIONS

Mix sugar, cornstarch, cinnamon, and nutmeg in a large pan. Add water and salt and mix well. Bring to a boil and cook until thick and bubbly. Remove from heat and add lemon juice and food coloring.

Sterilize canning jars, lids, and rings by boiling them in a large pot of water.

Peel, core, and slice apples. Pack the sliced apples into hot canning jars, leaving a 1/2 inch of headspace.

Fill jars with hot syrup, and gently remove air bubbles with a knife.

Put lids on and process in a water bath canner for 20 minutes.

Hard Candy

INGREDIENTS

cooking spray

3 ¾ cups white sugar

1 ½ cups light corn syrup

1 cup water

1 tablespoon orange, or other flavored extract

½ teaspoon food coloring (Optional)

¼ cup confectioners' sugar for dusting

INSTRUCTIONS

Grease a cookie sheet with cooking spray.

Stir white sugar, corn syrup, and water together in a medium saucepan. Cook, stirring, over medium heat until sugar dissolves, then bring to a boil.

Without stirring, heat to 300 to 310 degrees F (149 to 154 degrees C), or until a small amount of syrup dropped into cold water forms hard, brittle threads.

Remove from the heat and stir in flavored extract and food coloring. Pour onto the prepared cookie sheet. Dust top with confectioners' sugar.

Let cool until hardened, about 15 minutes. Break into about 36 pieces and store in an airtight container.

Easy Corn on the Cob

INGREDIENTS

2 tablespoons white sugar

1 tablespoon lemon juice

6 ears corn on the cob, husks and silk removed

INSTRUCTIONS

Fill a large pot about 3/4 full of water and bring to a boil. Stir in sugar and lemon juice until sugar is dissolved.

Gently place ears of corn into boiling water, cover the pot, turn off the heat, and let corn cook in the hot water until tender, about 10 minutes.

Homemade Applesauce

INGREDIENTS

4 apples - peeled, cored and chopped

¾ cup water

¼ cup white sugar

½ teaspoon ground cinnamon

INSTRUCTIONS

Combine apples, water, sugar, and cinnamon in a saucepan; cover and cook over medium heat until apples are soft, about 15 to 20 minutes.

Allow apple mixture to cool, then mash with a fork or potato masher until it is the consistency you like.

Classic Spanish Rice

INGREDIENTS

2 tablespoons oil

2 tablespoons chopped onion

1 ½ cups uncooked white rice

2 cups chicken broth

1 cup picante sauce

INSTRUCTIONS

Heat oil in a large, heavy skillet over medium heat. Add onion; cook and stir until tender, about 5 minutes.

Add rice; cook and stir until rice begins to turn golden brown. Stir in chicken broth and picante sauce. Reduce heat, cover, and simmer until liquid has been absorbed, about 15 to 20 minutes.

Tasty Za'atar Carrots and Lentils

INGREDIENTS

1 lb. multicolor baby carrots, peeled, trimmed, and halved lengthwise

1 tablespoon pure maple syrup

2 teaspoons salt-free za'atar seasoning

1⅔ cups dry French lentils, rinsed and drained

2 cups low-sodium vegetable broth

½ cup chopped onion

2 tablespoons no-salt-added tomato paste

2 sprigs fresh thyme

¾ cup pitted Castelvetrano olives, coarsely chopped

¼ cup golden raisins

¼ cup chopped garlic scapes or scallions

1 teaspoon lemon zest

Lemon wedges

INSTRUCTIONS

In an extra-large nonstick skillet combine carrots, maple syrup, za'atar seasoning, and ¼ cup water. Cover and cook over medium 14 to 16 minutes or until carrots are tender. Uncover; cook 1 minute more or until carrots are glazed and golden, stirring occasionally. Remove carrots from skillet.

In the same skillet combine the lentils and the next four ingredients (through thyme) plus 1½ cups water. Bring to boiling; reduce heat. Cover and simmer 25 to 30 minutes or until lentils are tender. Remove and discard thyme.

Stir in olives, raisins, garlic scapes, and lemon zest. Place carrots on top. Cover and heat through. If you like, sprinkle with additional za'atar seasoning. Serve with lemon wedges.

Savory Lavender and Lemon Tart

INGREDIENTS

1½ cups rolled oats

¼ cup sliced almonds, toasted

1 tablespoon poppy seeds

½ cup mashed banana (1 medium)

1½ cups unsweetened, unflavored plant-based milk

1¼ teaspoons agar powder

1 teaspoon chopped dried lavender

2 teaspoons lemon zest

½ cup lemon juice

⅓ cup pure maple syrup

¼ teaspoon ground turmeric

¼ teaspoon sea salt

Lemon slices

INSTRUCTIONS

Preheat oven to 350°F. For crust, in a food processor combine oats, almonds, and poppy seeds; pulse until well blended. Add banana; pulse until mixture holds together. With damp hands, press mixture over bottom and up sides of a 9-inch nonstick tart pan with a removable bottom. Bake 20 minutes or until dry and light brown. Remove from oven and let cool.

For filling, measure milk in a measuring cup; transfer 2 tablespoons of the milk to a small bowl. Add agar powder to the 2 tablespoons milk and stir to make a paste.

In a medium saucepan heat the remaining milk and the lavender over medium until it begins to steam. Whisk in agar mixture. Bring to boiling over medium; reduce heat. Simmer, uncovered, 5 minutes, stirring occasionally. Transfer mixture to a medium bowl. Let cool 30 minutes or until just warm to the touch.

Stir the next five ingredients (through salt) into warm milk mixture. Pour filling into crust. Chill at least 4 hours or overnight. Sprinkle with additional lavender and serve with lemon slices.

Sweet Crispy Air-Fried Tofu with Brown Rice Noodles

INGREDIENTS

2 medium pitted Medjool dates

¼ cup natural creamy peanut butter

5 tablespoons coconut aminos

1 tablespoon lime juice

⅛ teaspoon cayenne pepper (plus ¼ teaspoon, optional)

1 14- to 16-oz. package extra-firm tofu

2 tablespoons cornstarch

½ teaspoon ground ginger

4 scallions

1 stalk fresh lemongrass, trimmed and thinly sliced (2 tablespoons)

1 to 2 medium fresh Thai chiles or serrano chiles, stemmed and thinly sliced

2 medium heads baby bok choy, trimmed and quartered lengthwise

10 oz. dry brown rice pad Thai noodles, cooked according to package directions

¼ cup low-sodium vegetable broth

½ cup fresh broccoli sprouts (optional)

Lime wedges (optional)

INSTRUCTIONS

For peanut sauce, in a blender combine the dates and ½ cup boiling water. Cover and let stand 15 minutes. Add peanut butter, 2 tablespoons of the coconut aminos, the lime juice, and ⅛ teaspoon cayenne pepper. Cover and blend until smooth, scraping sides of blender as needed. Transfer sauce to a small saucepan.

Place tofu between folded paper towels. Top with a plate and a heavy can of food. Let stand 15 minutes. Cut tofu into 1-inch cubes and place in a medium bowl. Add 2 tablespoons of the coconut aminos; toss to coat. Let rest 5 minutes; toss again until all the liquid is absorbed. In a small bowl stir together cornstarch, ginger, and cayenne pepper (if using). Sprinkle half the cornstarch mixture over tofu; toss gently to coat. Sprinkle the remaining cornstarch mixture over tofu; toss gently.

Preheat air fryer to 400°F. Arrange tofu in a single layer in air-fryer basket. Air-fry 8 to 10 minutes or until tofu is golden brown.

Meanwhile, thickly slice scallion whites and bias-slice greens. In a large skillet or wok cook scallion whites, lemongrass, and chile slices over medium 1 to 2 minutes or until fragrant, stirring frequently and adding water, 1 to 2 tablespoons at a time, as needed to prevent sticking.

Add bok choy to skillet. Cook 6 to 8 minutes more or until lightly wilted, adding water, 1 to 2 tablespoons. at a time, as needed to prevent sticking. Heat Peanut Sauce over medium-low 2 to 3 minutes or until heated through, whisking frequently.

In a medium bowl combine cooked noodles, vegetable broth, the remaining 1 tablespoon coconut aminos, and half of the peanut sauce; toss to combine. Add a little water if noodles are sticking together.

Divide noodles, vegetables, and tofu among four shallow bowls. Drizzle with the remaining peanut sauce. Top with scallion greens. If you like, top with broccoli sprouts and serve with lime wedges.

Gluten-Free Crepes

INGREDIENTS

2 cups chickpea flour

½ cup tapioca flour

Pinch of sea salt

2½ cups unsweetened, unflavored plant-based milk

½ cup + 2 tablespoons vegan gluten-free chocolate chips

2½ cups sliced fresh strawberries

INSTRUCTIONS

Sift flours and salt into a large bowl and whisk to combine. Add milk; whisk thoroughly to create a very thin, smooth batter. Let batter stand 2 minutes; whisk again to break up any lumps. Alternatively, make batter in a blender.

Heat a large nonstick skillet or griddle over medium-low. Pour slightly less than ½ cup batter into skillet. Use a batter spreader to evenly coat bottom of skillet with batter, or lift and tilt the skillet to spread batter. Cook 60 to 90 seconds or until the top is no longer shiny, then use a crepe turner or long, thin spatula to flip crepe.

Immediately sprinkle chocolate chips over half of the crepe, leaving a 1-inch border around edges. Cook 45 to 60 seconds more or until top looks dry on the second side. Lay ¼ cup sliced strawberries over chocolate. Fold crepe in half to cover fillings, then fold in half again. Repeat with remaining batter, chocolate chips, and strawberries.

Delicious Balsamic-Roasted Delicata Squash Salad

INGREDIENTS

2 lb. delicata squash, trimmed, sliced into ½-inch rings, seeds removed

⅔ cup balsamic vinegar

¼ cup lemon juice

2 tablespoons Dijon mustard

4 cups multicolor cherry tomatoes, halved

4 cups cooked tricolor quinoa, seasoned with sea salt and freshly ground black pepper

2 15-oz. cans no-salt-added cannellini beans, rinsed and drained (3 cups)

2 cups fresh basil leaves or baby arugula

4 cloves garlic, minced

½ teaspoon onion powder

INSTRUCTIONS

Preheat oven to 400°F. Line a 15x10- inch baking pan with parchment paper or a silicone baking mat. Place squash in a single layer in pan. In a small bowl whisk together balsamic vinegar, lemon juice, mustard, and ¼ cup water. Brush 2 tablespoons of the mixture over squash, reserving the remaining balsamic mixture for dressing. Roast squash 30 to 35 minutes or until tender. Cool in pan on a wire rack.

On a serving platter layer half each of the cooled squash, tomatoes, quinoa, beans, and basil. Repeat layers.

Whisk garlic and onion powder into the remaining balsamic mixture. Drizzle over salad.

Sweet and Spicy Air-Fried Brussels Sprouts

INGREDIENTS

½ lb. Brussels sprouts, trimmed and halved

3 tablespoons unseasoned brown rice vinegar

3 tablespoons pure maple syrup or brown rice syrup

1½ tablespoons Sriracha sauce

3 cloves garlic, minced

INSTRUCTIONS

Preheat air fryer to 375°F. In a large bowl toss sprouts with vinegar. Place sprouts in a single layer in air-fryer basket. (You may have to cook in batches.) Air-fry 15 minutes or until crisp and lightly browned.

Meanwhile, in a small saucepan combine maple syrup, sriracha, and garlic. Heat over medium-low for 2 minutes. In a serving bowl combine sprouts and syrup mixture. Toss to coat.

Wholesome Pinto Bean Spread

INGREDIENTS

1 cup peeled garlic cloves

1 pinch dried thyme

Sea salt, to taste

Freshly ground black pepper, to taste

2 15.5-oz. cans no-salt-added pinto beans (3 cups)

¼ cup lemon juice

1 teaspoon mild New Mexico red chile powder (optional)

INSTRUCTIONS

For Blackened Garlic, heat a small cast-iron skillet over high. Add garlic cloves to hot skillet. Cook 3 minutes or until garlic starts to blacken. Cook and stir 3 minutes more or until garlic is lightly blackened on all sides. Add dried thyme and a pinch each of sea salt and freshly ground black pepper; toss to coat. Transfer to a cutting board; let cool. Mince garlic.

Drain pinto beans, reserving liquid. Rinse and drain beans. If you like, reserve a few beans for garnish.

In a food processor combine beans and 3 tablespoons Blackened Garlic; process until smooth. Add lemon juice and chile powder (if using). Season with salt and black pepper. Process until creamy. (There should be no lumps.) Add reserved liquid from the pinto beans, 1 to 2 tablespoons at a time, as needed to reach desired texture. Top with reserved beans (if using) and additional chile powder. Serve Pinto Bean Spread immediately or store in an airtight container in the refrigerator up to 3 days. Store leftover Blackened Garlic in a separate airtight container in the refrigerator up to 4 days.

Kid-Friendly Rainbow Salad

INGREDIENTS

1½ teaspoons sea salt

1½ cups dry whole wheat couscous

3 medium Persian cucumbers, sliced (about 2 cups)

1 15-oz. can kidney beans, rinsed and drained (1½ cups)

1¼ cups fresh or thawed frozen yellow corn kernels

1 cup finely chopped red onion

2 medium red beets, peeled, quartered, and thinly sliced (1 cup)

1 cup cooked shelled edamame

½ cup finely chopped red bell pepper

½ cup finely chopped green bell pepper

½ cup finely chopped orange bell pepper

¼ cup orange juice

¼ cup pure maple syrup

2 tablespoons balsamic vinegar

1½ tablespoons lemon juice

2 teaspoons dried Italian seasoning, crushed

½ teaspoon freshly ground black pepper

½ teaspoon garlic powder

INSTRUCTIONS

In a medium saucepan combine 1½ cups water and ½ teaspoon of the salt. Bring to boiling; stir in couscous. Remove from heat and let stand, covered, 5 minutes. Spread couscous on a serving platter.

Arrange the next nine ingredients (through orange pepper) over couscous.

For dressing, in a jar combine the remaining ingredients and 1 teaspoon salt. Cover and shake well. Pour dressing over salad.

Kid-Friendly Edible Flower Salad

INGREDIENTS

3 cups baby lettuce leaves or other salad greens

1 cup finely chopped kale

½ cup shredded green cabbage

½ cup shredded red cabbage

¼ cup shredded carrot

½ cup sliced or chopped cucumber

½ cup chopped red bell pepper

½ cup sugar snap peas, trimmed and cut into thirds

¼ cup finely chopped red onion

¼ cup dried cranberries

¼ cup roasted pepitas

2 tablespoons fresh cilantro leaves

1 cup broccoli florets

6 to 8 nasturtiums, calendulas, violets, dandelions, or other edible flowers

½ cup pure maple syrup

¼ cup + 2 tablespoons Dijon or yellow mustard

2 tablespoons oil-free baba ghanoush or hummus

1½ tablespoon lemon juice

1½ teaspoons white wine vinegar

1½ teaspoons everything bagel seasoning

INSTRUCTIONS

In a large bowl combine the first nine ingredients (through cilantro); gently toss until mixed. Decorate the edges of the salad with broccoli and edible flowers.

For dressing, in a jar combine the remaining ingredients. Cover and shake well. Serve dressing on the side (kids may like dipping their broccoli "trees" into it), or drizzle it over salad just before serving.

CHAPTER VIII

BEFORE YOU LEAVE, A FINAL WORD!

Adopting a specialized diet for gallstone prevention and management has numerous benefits. Below are possible benefits you are sure to enjoy if you adopt a specialized diet:

- Reduced Symptoms: A well-planned diet can help alleviate the painful symptoms associated with gallstones, such as abdominal pain, nausea, and indigestion.

- Prevention: By avoiding certain foods and incorporating others, you can reduce the likelihood of gallstone formation.

- Overall Health: A diet aimed at preventing gallstones can also contribute to overall health and well-being, as it often includes nutrient-rich foods that support various bodily functions.

- Weight Management: Maintaining a healthy weight through a balanced diet can decrease the risk of gallstones, especially since obesity is a known risk factor.